CHAIR YOGA FOR SENIORS OVER 70

The Comprehensive Guide For Older Men And Women To Lose Weight, Prevent Aging And Enhance Strength, Flexibility, Mobility And Balance With Easy Daily Workouts

Jared B. Graham

Table of Contents

INTRODUCTION

Meet Evelyn, a 72-year-old with a spirit as vibrant as the dawn but a body that didn't quite match her youthful zest. Like many seniors, Evelyn faced the all-too-common challenges of aging: joint pain, reduced mobility, and a creeping sense of isolation that often shadows the golden years. Activities that once brought joy, like gardening or long walks in the park, became sources of frustration rather than fulfillment.

Evelyn's discovery of chair yoga marked a turning point. This gentle form of exercise, designed with the limitations and needs of seniors in mind, became her gateway to reclaiming a sense of independence and well-being. Chair yoga, with its accessible poses and emphasis on mindfulness and breath control, offered Evelyn and others like her a solution to the problems that often accompany aging.

Through regular practice, Evelyn noticed a remarkable transformation. The stiffness that greeted her each morning began to ebb, replaced by a fluidity of movement she thought was lost to the past. Joint pain, a constant companion, diminished, allowing her to engage once again in the activities she loved but had set aside.

But the benefits of chair yoga extended beyond the physical. Evelyn found a new community among her fellow practitioners, combating the isolation that so often creeps into the lives of seniors. The focus on mindful breathing and meditation brought a sense of calm and clarity, reducing stress and enhancing her overall quality of life.

This guide, inspired by Evelyn's journey and the countless others who have discovered chair yoga as a lifeline in their later years, is more than just a collection of exercises. It's a roadmap to navigating the challenges of aging with grace, strength, and a renewed sense of vitality. Chair yoga has proven to be not just an activity but a transformative practice, offering solutions to the physical and emotional challenges that come with age.

Join us in exploring how chair yoga can be your ally in facing the golden years with optimism, health, and joy. Let's embark on this journey together, making every pose a step towards a fuller, more vibrant life.

CHAPTER 1

Benefits Of Chair Yoga For Seniors Over 70

1. Improved Flexibility: Regular chair yoga practice gently stretches the muscles and joints, leading to increased flexibility. This is crucial for seniors, as flexibility decreases with age, affecting the ease of performing daily activities.

2. Enhanced Strength: Chair yoga helps build strength in a safe and controlled manner, focusing on core muscles, arms, and legs. Stronger muscles contribute to better balance, which is essential for preventing falls.

3. Better Balance and Stability: By strengthening the core and improving flexibility, chair yoga enhances balance and stability. This reduces the risk of falls, a common concern for seniors, thereby promoting independence.

4. Joint Health: The gentle movements and poses in chair yoga can help alleviate joint discomfort by increasing circulation and reducing inflammation. This is particularly beneficial for those with arthritis.

5. Reduced Stress and Anxiety: Chair yoga incorporates breathing exercises and meditation, which can help lower stress levels and reduce anxiety. The focus on mindful breathing encourages a state of relaxation and well-being.

6. Improved Mental Clarity and Focus: The meditative aspects of chair yoga improve concentration and cognitive function. This can be especially valuable in combating age-related cognitive decline.

7. Increased Circulation: The physical activity involved in chair yoga helps boost circulation, ensuring that oxygen and nutrients are efficiently distributed throughout the body. Improved circulation supports heart health and aids in the healing process.

8. Pain Management: Regular practice can lead to pain reduction, especially in areas affected by chronic conditions such as lower back pain. This is achieved through the strengthening and stretching of muscles surrounding the problem areas.

9. Enhanced Respiratory Function: Breathing exercises in chair yoga improve lung capacity and respiratory function. This is crucial for seniors, especially those dealing with respiratory conditions or recovering from illnesses.

10. Improved Sleep Quality: Regular participation in chair yoga can lead to better sleep patterns. The relaxation techniques and stress reduction associated with yoga practice help in calming the mind and easing the transition into a restful sleep, which is often a challenge for seniors.

Safety Precautions And Guidelines Of Chair Yoga For Seniors Over 70

1. Consult with Healthcare Providers: Before starting any new exercise program, including chair yoga, seniors should consult with their healthcare providers, especially if they have any pre-existing health conditions or concerns.

2. Use a Stable Chair: Choose a sturdy chair without wheels that can support your weight comfortably. The chair should allow you to plant your feet firmly on the ground while seated, ensuring stability during poses.

3. Wear Appropriate Clothing: Wear comfortable, non-restrictive clothing that allows for a full range of motion. Also, practice barefoot or wear non-slip socks to prevent slipping.

4. Warm Up Properly: Begin each session with gentle warm-up exercises to prepare your body for more active poses. This can help reduce the risk of injury.

5. Understand Your Limits: Recognize your body's limits and avoid pushing yourself too hard. It's important to listen to your body and modify poses as needed to avoid strain or discomfort.

6. Maintain Proper Alignment: Pay close attention to your instructor's guidance on proper alignment and posture to ensure you're performing each pose safely and effectively.

7. Stay Hydrated: Keep water nearby and stay hydrated before, during, and after your chair yoga session, especially if you're practicing in a warm environment.

8. Avoid Holding Your Breath: Ensure you're breathing steadily and deeply throughout the practice. Holding your breath can increase blood pressure and stress on the body.

9. Use Props for Support: Don't hesitate to use props such as blocks, straps, or cushions to modify poses for comfort and support. These can help you maintain balance and alignment.

10. Practice Regularly but Don't Overdo It: Regular practice can help improve strength, flexibility, and balance over time, but it's important not to overdo it. Allow yourself rest days to recover and avoid fatigue or overexertion.

Essential Equipment Needed For Chair Yoga

1. Ergonomic Chair without Wheels: The chair is the foundation of your practice. Choose a sturdy, stable chair without wheels to prevent it from moving during exercises. It should have a comfortable seat and a supportive backrest. Ensure the chair is of a height that allows your feet to rest flat on the floor, with your knees and hips forming a 90-degree angle.

2. Yoga Mat: A yoga mat placed under the chair can prevent slipping, especially on hard or smooth surfaces. Additionally, if any part of the practice involves standing poses or floor work, the mat provides a cushioned, grippy surface.

3. Yoga Blocks: Yoga blocks are versatile accessories that can help modify poses to accommodate your flexibility level. They can be used to support your hands in standing poses or to reduce the stretch in seated poses, making the practice accessible and comfortable.

4. Yoga Strap: A strap can assist in stretches, helping you maintain proper alignment without straining. It's especially useful for leg and shoulder stretches, allowing you to gently deepen the stretch without compromising your posture.

5. Cushions and Pillows: Cushions and pillows can be used to modify the seat height if the chair is too low or to provide additional support and comfort, particularly for the back or to sit on for added hip elevation.

6. Resistance Bands: For those looking to incorporate strength training into their chair yoga routine, resistance bands are a great tool. They can be used for various arm and leg exercises, offering adjustable resistance based on your strength level.

7. Comfortable, Breathable Clothing: While technically not "equipment," the right clothing can significantly affect your practice. Wear garments that allow you to move freely and don't restrict your range of motion.

8. Stable Footwear or Barefoot: Depending on your practice environment and personal preference, you might opt for barefoot to enhance your grip and proprioception or wear stable, non-slip shoes or socks for additional support and safety.

9. Blanket: A folded blanket can serve multiple purposes: providing warmth, acting as a prop for seated poses, or offering additional cushioning for knees or hips during certain poses.

10. Water Bottle: Hydration is key to any physical activity, including chair yoga. Keep a water bottle within reach to ensure you stay hydrated throughout your practice.

CHAPTER 2

Breathing Techniques For Relaxation And Vitality

1. Diaphragmatic Breathing (Belly Breathing):

- How to Do It: Sit or lie down comfortably. Place one hand on your belly and the other on your chest. Inhale deeply through your nose, allowing your belly to push your hand out. Your chest should remain relatively still. Exhale through pursed lips as if whistling, feeling the hand on your belly go in, and use it to gently push all the air out.

- Benefits: This technique promotes deep, full breaths, which can reduce stress, lower heart rate, and help with overall relaxation.

2. 4-7-8 Breathing:

- How to Do It: Sit or lie in a comfortable position. Close your mouth and inhale quietly through your nose to a mental count of four. Hold your breath for a count of seven. Exhale completely through your mouth, making a whoosh sound, to a count of eight.

- Benefits: The 4-7-8 breathing technique is a natural tranquilizer for the nervous system. It can help reduce anxiety, improve sleep, and manage stress responses.

3. Box Breathing (Square Breathing):

- How to Do It: Inhale to a count of four, hold your breath for a count of four, exhale for a count of four, and then hold again for a count of four. This creates a "box" or "square" pattern in your breathing.

- Benefits: Box breathing is used for concentration and alertness, making it beneficial for moments requiring focus or calmness. It can also be a powerful stress reliever.

4. Alternate Nostril Breathing (Nadi Shodhana):

- How to Do It: Sit in a comfortable position. Hold your right thumb over your right nostril and inhale deeply through your left nostril. At the peak of inhalation, close off the left nostril with your ring finger, then exhale through the right nostril. Continue this pattern, inhaling through the right nostril, closing it off, and exhaling through the left.

- Benefits: This technique helps to balance the left and right hemispheres of the brain, reduce stress, and enhance cardiovascular function. It's known for its ability to refresh and revitalize the body.

5. Bee Breath (Bhramari Pranayama):

- How to Do It: Close your ears with your thumbs and place your fingers over your eyes. Inhale deeply through your nose, then, keeping your mouth closed, exhale while making a humming sound like a bee.

- Benefits: Bee breath is effective for calming the mind, relieving stress and anxiety, and improving concentration. It's particularly useful for soothing the nervous system before sleep.

WARM UP EXERCISES

1. Neck Rolls

- **Starting Position:** Sit comfortably in your chair with your spine straight and feet flat on the ground.

- **Steps:** Lower your chin to your chest, then slowly roll your head to the right, bringing your ear towards your shoulder. Gently roll your head back, then to the left side, completing a full circle. Repeat in the opposite direction.

- **Repetitions:** 3-5 times in each direction.

- **Purpose:** To release tension in the neck and improve flexibility.

2. Shoulder Rolls

- **Starting Position:** Sit upright with your feet planted firmly on the floor, hands resting on your thighs.

- **Steps:** Lift your shoulders up towards your ears, then roll them back, down, and forward in a circular motion.

- **Repetitions:** 5-10 times, then reverse the direction.

- **Purpose:** To reduce stiffness and increase mobility in the shoulders and upper back.

3. Seated Cat-Cow Stretch

- **Starting Position:** Sit on the edge of the chair with your feet flat on the ground, hands on your knees.

- **Steps:** Inhale and arch your back, tilting your pelvis forward while lifting your head and tailbone towards the ceiling (Cow). Exhale, round your spine, tuck your chin to your chest, and pull your belly in (Cat).

- **Repetitions:** 5-8 cycles.

- **Purpose:** To improve flexibility in the spine and relieve tension in the back.

4. Ankle Circles

- **Starting Position:** Sit upright with your feet flat on the ground. Extend one leg out in front of you, heel resting on the floor.

- **Steps:** Rotate your foot in a circular motion, moving only your ankle. Complete the circles in one direction, then switch.

- **Repetitions:** 5-10 circles in each direction, then switch legs.

- **Purpose:** To increase circulation and mobility in the ankles, reducing the risk of swelling and stiffness.

5. Wrist Flex and Extend

- **Starting Position:** Sit with your spine straight, arms extended in front of you at shoulder height.

- **Steps:** Flex your wrists, pointing your fingers towards the ceiling, then extend, pointing them down towards the floor.

- **Repetitions:** 5-10 times.

- **Purpose:** To warm up and increase flexibility in the wrists, which is especially beneficial for those with arthritis or wrist stiffness.

FUNDAMENTAL CHAIR YOGA POSES

1. Seated Mountain Pose (Tadasana)

- **Starting Position:** Sit upright towards the front edge of the chair, feet flat on the ground, hands resting on your thighs.

- **Steps:** Inhale and extend your spine tall, imagining a string pulling you up from the crown of your head. Engage your abdominal muscles slightly. As you exhale, roll your shoulders down and back, palms facing forward to open the chest.

- **Repetitions:** Hold for 3-5 breaths.

- **Purpose:** To improve posture, strengthen the spine, and create a sense of groundedness.

2. Seated Forward Bend (Paschimottanasana)

- **Starting Position:** Sit with your legs together, extended in front of you on the ground or on another chair for support, spine straight.

- **Steps:** Inhale and extend your arms overhead, lengthening your spine. As you exhale, hinge at the hips and bend forward, reaching towards your toes. Keep your back straight.

- **Repetitions:** Hold for 3-5 breaths, then release and repeat 2-3 times.

- **Purpose:** To stretch the spine and hamstrings, improve digestion, and calm the mind.

3. Chair Pigeon Pose (Eka Pada Rajakapotasana)

- **Starting Position:** Sit upright with your feet flat on the floor.

- **Steps:** Lift your right leg and place your right ankle on your left knee, keeping your right knee open to the side. Inhale and lengthen your spine. Exhale and gently lean forward from your hips, maintaining a straight back, to deepen the stretch.

- **Repetitions:** Hold for 3-5 breaths, then switch legs and repeat.

- **Purpose:** To open the hips, stretch the thighs and glutes, and alleviate lower back tension.

4. Seated Twists

- **Starting Position:** Sit upright in the chair, feet flat on the ground.

- **Steps:** Place your right hand on the back of the chair. Inhale and lengthen your spine. As you exhale, gently twist your torso to the right, using your hand on the chair for support. Keep your hips facing forward.

- **Repetitions:** Hold for 3-5 breaths, then gently return to center and repeat on the opposite side.

- **Purpose:** To improve spinal mobility, stimulate digestion, and relieve stress.

CHAPTER 3

STRENGTH AND STABILITY EXERCISES

1. Chair Squats

- **Starting Position:** Stand in front of a chair with your feet hip-width apart, toes pointing forward.

- **Steps:** Extend your arms in front of you for balance. Slowly bend your knees and lower your body towards the chair as if you are going to sit down, but stop just before touching it, then stand back up.

- **Repetitions:** 8-10 times.

- **Purpose:** To strengthen the thighs, buttocks, and core, improving balance and stability.

2. Seated Leg Lifts

- **Starting Position:** Sit upright in the chair with feet flat on the ground and hands resting on the sides of the chair for support.

- **Steps:** Lift one leg straight out in front of you as high as comfortable, keeping the knee straight. Hold for a moment, then lower it back down. Repeat with the other leg.

- **Repetitions:** 8-10 times on each leg.

- **Purpose:** To strengthen the quadriceps and improve hip flexibility, contributing to better balance and mobility.

3. Seated Marching

- **Starting Position:** Sit upright with your feet flat on the floor and hands on your thighs or holding onto the sides of the chair.

- **Steps:** Lift your right knee towards your chest as high as comfortably possible, then place it back down. Repeat with your left knee, alternating in a marching motion.

- **Repetitions:** 15-20 times, alternating legs.

- **Purpose:** To strengthen the hip flexors and core muscles, enhancing stability and coordination.

4. Chair Supported Side Leg Raises

- **Starting Position:** Stand beside the chair, holding onto the back of the chair for support, feet slightly apart.

- **Steps:** Keeping your body straight, slowly lift your leg away from your body to the side as high as comfortable, then lower it back down with control. Repeat on the other side.

- **Repetitions:** 8-10 times on each side.

- **Purpose:** To strengthen the abductor muscles of the hips, enhancing lateral stability and reducing the risk of falls.

5. Toe Taps

- **Starting Position:** Sit upright in the chair with feet flat on the ground.

- **Steps:** Lift the toes of one foot as high as you can while keeping your heel on the ground, then lower them back down. Repeat with the other foot.

- **Repetitions:** 10-15 times on each foot.

- **Purpose:** To improve the strength and flexibility of the lower leg muscles, particularly the shin muscles, which are important for walking stability and preventing trips.

6. Seated Knee Extensions

- **Starting Position:** Sit upright in the chair with feet flat on the ground.

- **Steps:** Lift one foot off the floor and extend your leg in front of you as straight as possible, then flex your foot to emphasize the stretch in your calf and hamstring. Return to the starting position and repeat with the other leg.

- **Repetitions:** 8-10 times per leg.

- **Purpose:** To strengthen the quadriceps and improve knee joint stability, aiding in activities that require knee use like walking and climbing stairs.

7. Chair Push-ups

- **Starting Position:** Sit at the edge of the chair with your hands placed on either side of your hips, fingers pointing towards the front.

- **Steps:** Push down into the chair with your hands to lift your body slightly off the seat, then lower yourself back down. Keep your back straight and core engaged.

- **Repetitions:** 8-10 times.

- **Purpose:** To strengthen the arms, shoulders, and chest, enhancing upper body stability and functional strength for daily tasks.

8. Seated Tummy Twists

- **Starting Position:** Sit upright in the chair, feet flat on the ground, and place your hands behind your head with elbows wide.

- **Steps:** Gently twist your torso to the right, aiming to bring your left elbow towards your right knee without moving your hips. Return to center and repeat on the opposite side.

- **Repetitions:** 8-10 times per side.

- **Purpose:** To strengthen the core muscles, particularly the obliques, which are essential for torsional stability and preventing lower back pain.

9. Ankle Flex and Point

- **Starting Position:** Sit upright with your feet slightly off the ground or resting on the edge of another chair.

- **Steps:** Flex your feet, pulling the toes towards you, then point your toes away from you.

- **Repetitions:** 10-15 times.

- **Purpose:** To improve the flexibility and strength of the ankle and calf muscles, contributing to better balance and preventing ankle stiffness.

10. Seated Hip Openers

- **Starting Position:** Sit upright in the chair, feet flat on the ground.

- **Steps:** Place one foot over the opposite knee, forming a figure-4 shape with your legs. Gently press down on the raised knee for a deeper hip stretch. Maintain an upright posture to enhance the stretch.

- **Repetitions:** Hold for 15-30 seconds per side.

- **Purpose:** To open up the hips and stretch the glutes and inner thigh muscles, improving hip mobility and reducing discomfort from sitting.

FLEXIBILITY AND MOBILITY EXERCISES

1. Seated Side Stretch

- **Starting Position:** Sit upright in the chair, feet flat on the floor, and spine tall.

- **Steps:** Extend your right arm overhead and lean to the left side, gently stretching the right side of your body. Keep your left hand on your left thigh or the side of the chair for support. Return to the center and repeat on the other side.

- **Repetitions:** Hold for 3-5 breaths on each side.

- **Purpose:** To stretch the side body, improve lateral flexibility, and enhance intercostal muscle mobility, which can aid in deeper breathing.

2. Seated Forward Fold

- **Starting Position:** Sit with your legs slightly apart, feet flat on the ground, and spine straight.

- **Steps:** Inhale and lengthen your spine. As you exhale, hinge at the hips and fold forward, allowing your hands to rest on your shins, ankles, or the floor. Let your head hang gently to relax your neck.

- **Repetitions:** Hold for 5-8 breaths, gently come back up, and repeat 2-3 times.

- **Purpose:** To stretch the back and hamstrings, increase spinal flexibility, and promote circulation to the upper body.

3. Seated Spinal Twist

- **Starting Position:** Sit upright in the chair, feet flat on the ground.

- **Steps:** Place your right hand on the back of the chair. Use your left hand on your right knee as leverage to gently twist your torso to the right. Keep your spine tall and gaze over your right shoulder. Return to center and repeat on the opposite side.

- **Repetitions:** Hold for 3-5 breaths on each side.

- **Purpose:** To increase spinal mobility, stimulate digestion, and relieve tension in the back.

4. Seated Hamstring Stretch

- **Starting Position:** Sit on the edge of the chair and extend one leg forward, heel on the ground, toe pointing up.

- **Steps:** Keeping your back straight, gently lean forward from the hips towards your extended leg until you feel a stretch in the back of your thigh. Hold, then return to the starting position and switch legs.

- **Repetitions:** Hold for 5-8 breaths on each leg.

- **Purpose:** To stretch the hamstrings and calves, improving leg flexibility and reducing the risk of back pain.

5. Seated Ankle Rolls

- **Starting Position:** Sit upright with one leg extended straight, foot off the ground, or resting on the edge of another chair.

- **Steps:** Rotate your ankle in a circular motion, first clockwise, then counter-clockwise. Focus on making smooth, complete circles to maximize the range of motion.

- **Repetitions:** 5-10 circles in each direction per ankle.

- **Purpose:** To improve ankle mobility and circulation, reducing stiffness and aiding in balance and walking.

6. Wrist and Finger Stretches

- **Starting Position:** Sit upright in your chair, arms extended forward at shoulder height.

- **Steps:** Spread your fingers wide, then make a fist. Next, bend your wrists down and then up. After several repetitions, circle your wrists in both directions.

- **Repetitions:** 5-10 times for each movement.

- **Purpose:** To increase flexibility and reduce stiffness in the wrists and fingers, beneficial for daily activities and alleviating symptoms of arthritis.

7. Neck Side Stretch

- **Starting Position:** Sit upright in the chair with your feet flat on the ground and hands resting on your lap.

- **Steps:** Gently tilt your head to one side, bringing your ear closer to the shoulder until you feel a stretch on the opposite side of your neck. Hold, then slowly return to the starting position and repeat on the other side.

- **Repetitions:** Hold for 3-5 breaths on each side.

- **Purpose:** To relieve tension in the neck muscles, enhance neck mobility, and improve posture.

8. Seated Eagle Arms

- **Starting Position:** Sit upright in the chair with your feet flat on the ground.

- **Steps:** Extend your arms straight in front of you at shoulder height. Cross your right arm over the left at the elbows, then bend the elbows to bring your palms to touch or get as close as possible. Lift your elbows while dropping your shoulders away from your ears. Hold, then unwind and repeat with the left arm over the right.

- **Repetitions:** Hold for 3-5 breaths on each side.

- **Purpose:** To stretch the shoulders and upper back, improve arm mobility, and reduce tension in the upper body.

9. Seated Hip and Thigh Stretch

- **Starting Position:** Sit upright towards the front edge of the chair, feet flat on the ground.

- **Steps:** Place your right ankle on your left knee, creating a figure-four shape. Keeping your back straight, gently lean forward from your hips until you feel a stretch in your right hip and thigh. Hold, then slowly return to the starting position and switch sides.

- **Repetitions:** Hold for 5-8 breaths on each side.

- **Purpose:** To open up the hips and stretch the glutes and piriformis, which can help relieve lower back and hip pain.

10. Seated Calf Stretch

- **Starting Position:** Sit towards the edge of the chair with one-foot flat on the ground and the other extended forward, heel on the ground and toe pointing up.

- **Steps:** Lean forward slightly from the hips, keeping your back straight, until you feel a stretch in the calf of the extended leg. Hold, then switch legs.

- **Repetitions:** Hold for 5-8 breaths per leg.

- **Purpose:** To stretch the calf muscles, improve lower leg mobility, and promote circulation, which is especially important for seniors to reduce the risk of peripheral vascular issues.

BALANCE AND COORDINATION EXERCISES

1. Seated Toe Taps

- **Starting Position:** Sit upright in the chair, feet flat on the floor, hands on your thighs.

- **Steps:** Extend one leg at a time, tapping the toe on the floor in front of you, then lift and return to starting position. Alternate legs with each tap.

- **Repetitions:** 10-15 taps per leg.

- **Purpose:** To improve coordination and strengthen the leg muscles, aiding in balance and walking stability.

2. Heel Raises

- **Starting Position:** Sit upright with your feet flat on the ground, holding onto the sides of the chair for support.

- **Steps:** Slowly lift both heels off the ground as high as you can, coming onto your toes, then lower them back down.

- **Repetitions:** 10-15 times.

- **Purpose:** To strengthen the calf muscles and improve balance by encouraging weight shifting and control.

3. Seated Marching

- **Starting Position:** Sit upright in the chair with your feet flat on the floor and hands resting on your thighs or holding onto the sides of the chair.

- **Steps:** Lift one knee towards your chest as high as comfortably possible, then place it back down. Alternate knees in a marching motion.

- **Repetitions:** 15-20 times, alternating legs.

- **Purpose:** To enhance coordination and strengthen the hip flexors and core, contributing to better balance and stability.

4. Single-Leg Extensions

- **Starting Position:** Sit upright in the chair, feet flat on the floor, hands on your thighs or holding onto the sides of the chair for support.

- **Steps:** Extend one leg out in front of you, keeping it as straight as possible. Hold the position for a few seconds, then lower it back down. Repeat with the other leg.

- **Repetitions:** 8-10 times per leg.

- **Purpose:** To improve leg strength and stability, enhancing balance while standing or walking.

5. Chair Stand

- **Starting Position:** Sit in the middle of the chair with your feet flat on the floor, slightly apart, and lean slightly forward.

- **Steps:** Cross your arms over your chest or place them on the opposite shoulders. Using your leg muscles, stand up slowly, then sit back down with control.

- **Repetitions:** 5-10 times.

- **Purpose:** To strengthen the thighs and buttocks, improve core stability, and enhance coordination and balance during transitions from sitting to standing.

6. Side Leg Raises

- **Starting Position:** Sit upright in the chair, holding onto the sides for support.

- **Steps:** Extend one leg out to the side as far as comfortably possible, keeping your foot flexed and the leg straight. Hold for a few seconds, then slowly bring it back to the starting position. Repeat on the other side.

- **Repetitions:** 8-10 times per leg.

- **Purpose:** To strengthen the abductor muscles and improve hip stability, aiding in balance and reducing the risk of sideways falls.

7. Seated "Tree Pose"

- **Starting Position:** Sit upright in the chair, feet flat on the floor.

- **Steps:** Place the sole of your right foot on the inner left thigh or calf (avoid the knee joint), mimicking the tree pose's leg position. Press your foot against the thigh and the thigh against the foot for stability. Hold your hands in prayer position in front of your chest or raise them above your head for more challenge.

- **Repetitions:** Hold for 3-5 breaths, then switch sides.

- **Purpose:** To enhance balance and coordination while strengthening the thighs and ankles. This pose also promotes concentration and focus.

8. Forward Toe Taps

- **Starting Position:** Stand behind the chair, lightly holding onto the back of the chair for support.

- **Steps:** Lift one foot and tap the toe a few inches in front of you, then bring it back. Alternate feet with each tap, maintaining a slow and controlled movement.

- **Repetitions:** 10-15 taps per foot.

- **Purpose:** To improve dynamic balance and coordination while engaging the core and leg muscles, essential for walking and stair climbing.

9. Backward Leg Lifts

- **Starting Position:** Stand behind the chair, hands lightly resting on the back of the chair for support.

- **Steps:** Gently lift one leg straight back without bending your knee or leaning forward. Hold for a moment, then lower it with control. Repeat on the other side.

- **Repetitions:** 8-10 times per leg.

- **Purpose:** To strengthen the glutes and lower back, improving postural stability and reducing the risk of falls by enhancing rear awareness.

10. Seated Heel-Toe Rock

- **Starting Position:** Sit upright in the chair, feet flat on the floor.

- **Steps:** Lift your heels high, coming onto your toes, then rock back onto your heels, lifting your toes off the floor. Continue this rocking motion smoothly.

- **Repetitions:** 10-15 times.

- **Purpose:** To stimulate the muscles and nerves in the feet and lower legs, improving proprioception (body position awareness) and aiding in balance during walking movements.

EXERCISES FOR IMPROVING SLEEP: RELAXING POSES AND TECHNIQUES

1. Seated Forward Bend (Paschimottanasana)

- **Starting Position:** Sit at the edge of the chair with legs extended forward, feet slightly apart.
- **Steps:** Inhale and extend your arms overhead to lengthen the spine. As you exhale, hinge at the hips to lean forward, reaching your hands towards your toes. Allow your head to hang gently, and focus on relaxing into the pose with each exhale.
- **Repetitions:** Hold for 5-8 breaths, gently come back up, and repeat if desired.
- **Purpose:** To calm the mind, relieve stress, and stretch the spine and hamstrings, facilitating relaxation and preparing the body for rest.

2. Seated Spinal Twist

- **Starting Position:** Sit upright in the chair, feet flat on the ground.

- **Steps:** Place your right hand on the back of the chair. Use your left hand on your right knee as leverage to gently twist your torso to the right. Keep your spine tall and gaze over your right shoulder. Return to center and repeat on the opposite side.

- **Repetitions:** Hold for 3-5 breaths on each side.

- **Purpose:** To release tension in the spine, detoxify the internal organs, and promote relaxation, helping to prepare the body for sleep.

3. Seated Extended Leg Pose

- **Starting Position:** Sit upright in the chair, extend one leg out straight in front of you, resting the heel on the floor with the toe pointed upward.

- **Steps:** Inhale and reach your arms up to lengthen the spine. As you exhale, hinge at the hips to lean forward slightly, reaching towards your extended foot. Hold the pose and focus on deep, relaxing breaths.

- **Repetitions:** Hold for 5-8 breaths, then switch legs.

- **Purpose:** To stretch the legs and lower back, reducing physical tension that can hinder sleep, while encouraging a calming effect on the mind.

4. Chair Pigeon Pose

- **Starting Position:** Sit upright in the chair, feet flat on the floor.

- **Steps:** Place your right ankle on your left knee, forming a figure-4 shape. Keep your back straight and gently lean forward to increase the stretch if needed. Focus on relaxing breaths.

- **Repetitions:** Hold for 5-8 breaths, then switch sides.

- **Purpose:** To open the hips and relieve tension in the lower body, promoting relaxation and reducing discomfort that may impair sleep quality.

5. Seated Savasana with Guided Relaxation

- **Starting Position:** Sit comfortably in your chair, hands resting on your lap or thighs, palms up or down based on comfort.

- **Steps:** Close your eyes and take deep breaths, inhaling through the nose and exhaling through the mouth. Starting from the top of your head, mentally scan down through your body, consciously relaxing each part until you reach your feet. Continue with deep, slow breaths.

- **Repetitions:** Spend 5-10 minutes in this state of relaxation.

- **Purpose:** To reduce mental stress and physical tension throughout the body, creating a state of deep relaxation that can ease the transition into sleep.

EXERCISES FOR JOINT HEALTH: MOVEMENTS TO EASE ARTHRITIS

1. Wrist Circles

- **Starting Position:** Sit upright in your chair with your feet flat on the floor. Extend your arms forward at shoulder height.

- **Steps:** Open your hands wide, then close them into fists. Slowly rotate your wrists in a circular motion, first clockwise, then counterclockwise.

- **Repetitions:** 5-10 circles in each direction.

- **Purpose:** To increase mobility and circulation in the wrists, reducing stiffness and discomfort associated with arthritis.

2. Ankle Pumps

- **Starting Position:** Sit upright with your back supported by the chair, legs extended out in front of you with heels on the floor.

- **Steps:** Point your toes away from you, stretching the front of the ankle, then flex your feet, bringing your toes towards you to stretch the calves and the back of the ankle.

- **Repetitions:** 10-15 times.

- **Purpose:** To improve ankle flexibility and circulation, helping to alleviate pain and stiffness in the ankle joints.

3. Seated Hip Openers

- **Starting Position:** Sit upright in the chair, feet flat on the ground.

- **Steps:** Place your right ankle on your left knee, forming a figure-4 shape. Keep your back straight and gently lean forward to increase the stretch if comfortable. Hold the stretch, then switch sides.

- **Repetitions:** Hold for 5-8 breaths on each side.

- **Purpose:** To gently stretch and open the hips, increasing mobility and easing discomfort in the hip joints.

4. Chair Cat-Cow Stretch

- **Starting Position:** Sit on the edge of the chair with your feet flat on the floor and hands on your knees.

- **Steps:** Inhale, arch your back, and look up, pushing your chest forward (Cow Pose). Exhale, round your spine, tucking your chin to your chest and pulling your belly in (Cat Pose).

- **Repetitions:** 5-8 cycles.

- **Purpose:** To increase flexibility and mobility in the spine, relieving stiffness and promoting circulation in the back.

5. Shoulder Rolls

- **Starting Position:** Sit upright in the chair with your feet flat on the ground and arms relaxed by your sides.

- **Steps:** Lift your shoulders towards your ears, then roll them back, down, and forward in a circular motion.

- **Repetitions:** 5-10 times in each direction.

- **Purpose:** To reduce shoulder stiffness and improve range of motion, beneficial for easing shoulder joint discomfort.

EXERCISES FOR MENTAL WELL-BEING: YOGA FOR ANXIETY AND DEPRESSION

1. Seated Deep Breathing (Pranayama)

- **Starting Position:** Sit comfortably in your chair with your back straight and feet flat on the floor.

- **Steps:** Place your hands on your abdomen. Inhale deeply through your nose, feeling your abdomen expand, then exhale slowly through your mouth, feeling your abdomen contract. Focus on making your breaths deep and slow.

- **Repetitions:** 5-10 deep breaths.

- **Purpose:** To reduce stress and anxiety, improve focus, and promote relaxation by activating the body's parasympathetic nervous system.

2. Gentle Seated Neck Stretches

- **Starting Position:** Sit upright in your chair, feet planted firmly on the ground.

- **Steps:** Gently tilt your head to one side, bringing your ear closer to your shoulder until you feel a stretch on the opposite side of your neck. Hold for a few breaths, then switch sides. Next, gently rotate your head to look over one shoulder, hold, then look over the other shoulder.

- **Repetitions:** Hold each stretch for 3-5 breaths on each side.

- **Purpose:** To release tension in the neck and shoulders, areas where emotional stress is often held, thereby reducing feelings of anxiety and depression.

3. Seated Mountain Pose with Overhead Stretch

- **Starting Position:** Sit upright with feet flat on the ground and arms at your sides.

- **Steps:** Inhale and slowly raise your arms overhead, palms facing each other. Clasp your hands together, stretching up as if trying to reach the ceiling, keeping your shoulders relaxed. Focus on your breath and the sensation of stretching.

- **Repetitions:** Hold for 3-5 breaths, then release and repeat 2-3 times.

- **Purpose:** To enhance body awareness and focus, reduce feelings of depression by opening up the chest and improving breathing, and bring a sense of balance and calm.

4. Seated Twist

- **Starting Position:** Sit upright in the center of the chair, feet flat on the floor.

- **Steps:** Place your right hand on the back of the chair. Inhale to lengthen your spine, and as you exhale, gently twist your torso to the right, keeping the hips facing forward. Hold for a few breaths, then return to center and repeat on the opposite side.

- **Repetitions:** Hold for 3-5 breaths on each side.

- **Purpose:** To release tension throughout the spine, stimulate digestion and circulation, and promote a sense of rejuvenation and clarity, which can help alleviate symptoms of anxiety and depression.

5. Gentle Seated Side Bends

- **Starting Position:** Sit upright in the chair, feet flat on the floor, and hands resting on the sides of the chair or in your lap.

- **Steps:** Inhale and gently raise your right arm overhead. On the exhale, lean to the left, stretching the right side of your body while keeping your sit bones firmly on the chair. Hold the stretch for a few breaths, focusing on the sensation of opening up the side of your body. Inhale to come back to center and repeat on the other side with your left arm.

- **Repetitions:** 3-5 times on each side.

- **Purpose:** To stretch and open the sides of the body, improving breathing capacity and promoting relaxation. Side bends can help alleviate feelings of tightness and restriction in the body that often accompany anxiety and depression, contributing to a sense of release and openness.

Mindfulness Practices for Daily Life

1. Mindful Breathing

- How to Practice: Find a comfortable seated position in a quiet space. Close your eyes and focus your attention on your breath. Notice the sensation of air entering and leaving your nostrils, the rise and fall of your chest or abdomen. When your mind wanders, gently bring your focus back to your breath.

- Purpose: To center your thoughts, calm the mind, and reduce stress. Mindful breathing can be a foundational practice for all mindfulness activities, helping to anchor you in the present moment.

2. Gratitude Journaling

- **How to Practice:** Each day, take a few moments to write down three things you are grateful for. These can be simple pleasures, people in your life, or positive experiences from the day. Reflect on why these things bring you joy or comfort.

- **Purpose:** To cultivate an attitude of gratitude, which has been shown to improve mental health, enhance well-being, and shift focus from negative to positive aspects of life.

3. Mindful Eating

- **How to Practice:** At meal times, focus fully on the experience of eating. Look at your food and appreciate its colors and textures. Chew slowly, savoring each bite, and notice the flavors and sensations in your mouth. Eat without distractions like TV or reading.

- **Purpose:** To enhance the enjoyment of food, improve digestion, and prevent overeating. Mindful eating encourages a deeper connection with your body's hunger and satiety signals.

4. Nature Connection

- **How to Practice:** Spend time in nature, whether it's a walk in the park, tending to a garden, or simply sitting outside. Observe the sights, sounds, and smells around you. Notice the details of the plants, the sky, and any animals you see.

- **Purpose:** To reduce feelings of loneliness and isolation, lower stress, and improve mood. Connecting with nature can foster a sense of belonging and peace.

5. Daily Affirmations

- **How to Practice:** Begin your day by stating positive affirmations aloud or silently to yourself. Choose affirmations that resonate with you, such as "I am at peace with myself," "I am grateful for another day," or "I am surrounded by love."

- **Purpose:** To set a positive tone for the day, boost self-esteem, and combat negative thought patterns. Affirmations can help create a more optimistic outlook and enhance overall well-being.

Guided Meditations for Peace and Clarity

1. Breath Awareness Meditation

Begin by finding a comfortable seated position. Close your eyes and take a moment to notice the natural rhythm of your breath without trying to change it.

- **Guidance:** Focus your attention on the sensation of air entering and exiting your nostrils. With each inhale, imagine drawing in peace and calm. With each exhale, visualize releasing any tension or stress. If your mind wanders, gently bring your focus back to your breath.

Gradually broaden your awareness beyond your breath to your entire body and then to the room around you. Open your eyes when you feel ready, carrying the sense of calm with you.

2. Body Scan for Relaxation

Lie down or sit comfortably. Close your eyes and take three deep breaths, releasing any obvious tension as you exhale.

- **Guidance:** Begin at the top of your head, slowly moving your attention down your body. Notice any areas of tension or discomfort, but instead of trying to change these sensations, simply observe them. As you scan down to your toes, imagine each part of your body relaxing and softening.

Once you've scanned your entire body, take a few moments to feel the collective weight of your relaxed body. Gently wiggle your fingers and toes, open your eyes, and return to your day, feeling refreshed.

3. Mindful Gratitude Meditation

Sit in a comfortable position, close your eyes, and focus on your breath, letting it flow naturally.

- **Guidance:** Think of three things you are grateful for. They can be as simple as the sun shining or having a friend who cares. For each one, pause and reflect on why you're thankful, imagining the feeling of gratitude filling your body with each breath.

Bring your focus back to the present moment, feeling enriched by the gratitude you've cultivated. When you're ready, open your eyes, carrying this sense of thankfulness with you.

4. Visualization for Peaceful Retreat

Find a comfortable seated or lying position. Close your eyes and breathe deeply, centering yourself.

- **Guidance:** Visualize a peaceful place, perhaps a quiet beach, a serene forest, or a cozy room. Explore this place in your mind, engaging all your senses—what do you see, hear, smell, and feel? Allow the tranquility of this place to envelop you, soothing any worries or stress.

Take a deep breath, and slowly bring your awareness back to the present. Gently open your eyes, feeling the peace from your visualization continue to calm your mind.

5. Loving-Kindness Meditation (Metta)

Begin in a comfortable seated position. Focus on your breath, letting it be gentle and relaxed.

- **Guidance:** First, direct loving-kindness towards yourself. You might silently say, "May I be happy, may I be healthy, may I live with ease." Then, gradually extend this loving-kindness outward to someone you love, someone you feel neutral about, someone you have difficulty with, and finally, to all beings everywhere.

As you conclude, take a moment to notice the warmth and openness in your heart. Open your eyes when you're ready, carrying forward this feeling of loving-kindness into your interactions.

Incorporating Yoga Principles Into Everyday Activities

Incorporating yoga principles into everyday activities can greatly enhance the quality of life for seniors over 70, making mundane tasks more meaningful and beneficial to overall well-being. Here's how seniors can weave yoga principles into their daily routines:

1. Mindfulness in Daily Tasks

Mindfulness, a core component of yoga, involves paying full attention to the present moment without judgment. Seniors can practice mindfulness during everyday activities such as eating, walking, or even during conversation. By fully engaging with the task at hand—notice the flavors and textures of your food, feel your feet touching the ground as you walk, listen intently to the person speaking—you cultivate a state of awareness that can lead to deeper appreciation and enjoyment of daily life.

2. Breath Awareness

Pranayama, or breath control, is another key aspect of yoga. Seniors can practice breath awareness throughout the day to calm the mind and reduce stress. For instance, while waiting in line or sitting through an appointment, focus on your breath. Take deep, slow breaths, inhaling fully and exhaling completely. This simple practice can help maintain calmness and clarity in potentially stressful situations.

3. Intention Setting

Yoga encourages setting an intention (Sankalpa) for your practice, which can be applied to daily life as well. Each morning, seniors can set a positive intention or goal for the day. It could be as simple as "Today, I will be kind to myself and others" or "I will find joy in small things." This practice helps focus the mind, guiding your actions and attitudes throughout the day.

4. Practicing Gratitude

Gratitude is deeply rooted in yoga philosophy, emphasizing the importance of being thankful for our experiences and what we have. Seniors can incorporate this principle by taking time each day to reflect on things they are grateful for. Keeping a gratitude journal or simply sharing thoughts of gratitude with a friend or family member can enhance feelings of well-being and contentment.

5. Applying Yoga Ethics in Interactions

Yoga's ethical guidelines, such as Ahimsa (non-violence) and Satya (truthfulness), can greatly influence how seniors interact with others and approach conflicts. Practicing kindness, patience, and honesty in dealings with friends, family, and caregivers fosters positive relationships and community connections. For example, approaching a disagreement with compassion and openness reflects the principle of Ahimsa, promoting harmony and understanding.

6. Physical Movement and Posture

Incorporating gentle yoga stretches and poses into routine activities can help maintain mobility, flexibility, and balance. For instance, performing a few seated stretches while watching TV or practicing balance exercises while holding onto a kitchen counter can integrate the benefits of yoga into daily life, contributing to physical health and reducing the risk of falls.

28-DAY CHAIR YOGA CHALLENGE FOR SENIORS OVER 70

Day 1: Introduction to Chair Yoga
1. Neck Rolls
2. Shoulder Rolls
3. Seated Mountain Pose (Tadasana)
4. Seated Deep Breathing (Pranayama)

Day 2: Focus on Flexibility
1. Seated Cat-Cow Stretch
2. Seated Forward Bend (Paschimottanasana)
3. Seated Spinal Twist
4. Gentle Seated Side Bends

Day 3: Building Strength
1. Chair Squats
2. Seated Leg Lifts
3. Seated Tummy Twists
4. Chair Push-ups

Day 4: Enhancing Stability and Balance
1. Seated Marching
2. Chair Supported Side Leg Raises
3. Seated "Tree Pose"
4. Heel Raises

Day 5: Mobility and Joint Health
1. Ankle Circles
2. Wrist Flex and Extend
3. Seated Hip Openers
4. Ankle Pumps

Day 6: Relaxation Techniques
1. Seated Extended Leg Pose
2. Chair Pigeon Pose
3. Seated Savasana with Guided Relaxation
4. Mindfulness Practices for Daily Life

Day 7: Mental Well-being
1. Gentle Seated Neck Stretches
2. Seated Mountain Pose with Overhead Stretch
3. Seated Twist
4. Guided Meditations for Peace and Clarity

Week 2: Deepening the Practice

Day 8: Core Stability and Balance
1. Toe Taps
2. Seated Knee Extensions
3. Seated Marching
4. Seated Hip and Thigh Stretch

Day 9: Flexibility and Mobility
1. Seated Side Stretch
2. Seated Forward Fold
3. Seated Ankle Rolls
4. Wrist and Finger Stretches

Day 10: Strengthening Exercises
1. Single-Leg Extensions
2. Side Leg Raises
3. Chair Stand
4. Seated "Tree Pose"

Day 11: Focus on Relaxation
1. Seated Forward Bend (Paschimottanasana)
2. Seated Spinal Twist
3. Seated Savasana with Guided Relaxation
4. Seated Deep Breathing (Pranayama)

Day 12: Enhancing Joint Health
1. Wrist Circles
2. Ankle Pumps
3. Chair Cat-Cow Stretch
4. Shoulder Rolls

Day 13: Improving Mental Well-being
1. Gentle Seated Neck Stretches
2. Seated Mountain Pose with Overhead Stretch
3. Seated Twist
4. Gentle Seated Side Bends

Day 14: Integration Day
1. Choose four favorite exercises from the past week.
2. Focus on breathing and gentle movements.
3. Reflect on the progress and how the body feels.
4. Practice mindfulness or guided meditation.

Week 3: Expanding Techniques

Day 15: Balance and Coordination
1. Seated Toe Taps
2. Heel Raises
3. Seated Marching
4. Forward Toe Taps

Day 16: Flexibility Focus
1. Seated Side Stretch
2. Seated Hamstring Stretch
3. Seated Calf Stretch
4. Neck Side Stretch

Day 17: Strength Building
1. Seated Leg Lifts
2. Chair Push-ups
3. Seated Tummy Twists
4. Chair Squats

Day 18: Relaxation and Mobility
1. Seated Extended Leg Pose
2. Chair Pigeon Pose
3. Seated Ankle Rolls
4. Wrist and Finger Stretches

Day 19: Joint Care

1. Ankle Circles
2. Seated Hip Openers
3. Wrist Flex and Extend
4. Seated Cat-Cow Stretch

Day 20: Mental and Emotional Well-being

1. Seated Deep Breathing (Pranayama)
2. Gentle Seated Neck Stretches
3. Seated Twist
4. Mindfulness Practices for Daily Life

Day 21: Personal Choice

1. Participants choose their four favorite exercises.
2. Encourage mixing different types of exercises (strength, flexibility, balance, relaxation).
3. Reflect on the benefits experienced so far.
4. Practice a longer session of guided meditation.

Week 4: Culmination and Maintenance

Day 22: Balancing Act

1. Backward Leg Lifts
2. Seated Heel-Toe Rock
3. Single-Leg Extensions
4. Side Leg Raises

Day 23: Flexibility and Strength

1. Seated Forward Fold
2. Seated Spinal Twist
3. Chair Squats
4. Seated Leg Lifts

Day 24: Enhancing Stability
1. Chair Supported Side Leg Raises
2. Seated Marching
3. Heel Raises
4. Seated "Tree Pose"

Day 25: Relaxation Techniques
1. Seated Savasana with Guided Relaxation
2. Seated Deep Breathing (Pranayama)
3. Seated Extended Leg Pose
4. Chair Pigeon Pose

Day 26: Joint Mobility
1. Ankle Pumps
2. Wrist Circles
3. Seated Hip Openers
4. Chair Cat-Cow Stretch

Day 27: Mental Clarity
1. Gentle Seated Neck Stretches
2. Seated Mountain Pose with Overhead Stretch
3. Seated Twist
4. Guided Meditations for Peace and Clarity

Day 28: Celebration of Practice
1. Participants select their top four exercises from the entire program.
2. Focus on mindful breathing and enjoying each movement.
3. Share experiences and reflect on the journey.
4. Close with a group guided meditation, focusing on gratitude and peace.

CONCLUSION

Chair yoga emerges as a beacon of hope and rejuvenation for seniors over 70, offering a pathway to enhanced well-being that is both accessible and profound. This gentle form of yoga, tailored to meet the unique needs of older adults, stands out as a holistic practice, nurturing the body, mind, and spirit in harmony. Through a series of seated and standing poses supported by a chair, it provides a safe and effective means to improve flexibility, strength, balance, and mental clarity, significantly enriching the quality of life in the golden years.

Importantly, chair yoga transcends the physical realm, touching upon the mental and emotional aspects of health. It introduces mindfulness and breath awareness into everyday activities, encouraging a deeper connection with the present moment and fostering a sense of peace and contentment. The practice of setting intentions and cultivating gratitude further enhances this journey, promoting positive outlooks and enriching relationships with oneself and others.

Moreover, chair yoga embodies the principle of adaptability, demonstrating that age and mobility limitations are not barriers to leading an active and fulfilling lifestyle. It invites seniors to explore their capabilities, gently pushing the boundaries of what they thought possible, and in doing so, redefines the aging process itself.

As we reflect on the myriad benefits chair yoga offers to seniors over 70, it's clear that this practice is more than just exercise, it's a celebration of life at any age. It encourages embracing each day with openness, joy, and gratitude, reminding us that it's never too late to start anew, to heal, and to thrive.

To the seniors contemplating this journey, let chair yoga be your guide to rediscovering vitality and serenity. Your golden years are a canvas awaiting your masterpiece, painted with the strokes of movement, mindfulness, and self-compassion. Begin this journey with an open heart, and watch as your life unfolds in vibrant hues of health and happiness.

BONUS: TOP 5 FACIAL EXERCISES FOR SENIORS OVER 70

1. The Forehead Smoother

- **Starting Position:** Sit or stand with a relaxed posture.

- **Steps:** Place both hands on your forehead facing inwards and spread your fingers out between the hairline and eyebrows. Gently sweep the fingers outwards across the forehead, applying light pressure to tighten the skin.

- **Repetitions:** Repeat 10 times.

- **Purpose:** Reduces the appearance of forehead wrinkles by relaxing and stretching the forehead muscles.

2. Eye Squeeze

- **Starting Position:** Sit or stand comfortably with your eyes open.
- **Steps:** Close your eyes tightly but without wrinkling your forehead. Hold this squeeze for 5-10 seconds, then relax and open your eyes.
- **Repetitions:** Do this 10 times.
- **Purpose:** Strengthens the muscles around the eyes to reduce crow's feet and under-eye sagging.

3. The Cheek Lifter

- **Starting Position:** Sit or stand with a relaxed posture.
- **Steps:** Open your mouth to form an "O". Pull your upper lip over your teeth, smile to lift cheek muscles up, then place your fingers lightly on the top part of your cheeks. Release the cheek muscles to lower them, and lift again. The resistance with your fingers helps improve muscle tone.
- **Repetitions:** Repeat 10-15 times.
- **Purpose:** Helps to firm and tone the cheeks, reducing sagging.

4. The Neck Lift

- **Starting Position:** Sit or stand with your back straight.
- **Steps:** Look straight ahead. Place your fingertips at the base of your neck and lightly pull the skin down as you tilt your head back. When your head is fully tilted back, pucker your lips as if you're trying to kiss the ceiling. Hold this position for 5-10 seconds.
- **Repetitions:** Repeat 5 times.
- **Purpose:** Strengthens the neck muscles and reduces the appearance of sagging and wrinkles in the neck area.

5. The Jaw and Face Toner

- **Starting Position:** Sit or stand with a relaxed posture.
- **Steps:** Close your mouth and press your lips together. Smile as wide as you can and hold for a second. Then, with your lips still pressed together, use your cheek muscles to push your lips up towards your nose. Hold this for 5 seconds.
- **Repetitions:** Do this 10 times.
- **Purpose:** Tones the cheeks and jawline, helping to reduce sagging and fine lines around the mouth.

Performing these facial exercises regularly can help seniors over 70 maintain a more youthful and vibrant appearance by improving muscle tone and skin elasticity. It's important to perform these exercises gently to avoid unnecessary strain and to achieve the best results over time.

BONUS: TOP 7 PELVIC FLOOR EXERCISES TO INCREASE SEXUAL PERFORMANCE

Pelvic floor exercises, often known as Kegel exercises, are vital for strengthening the muscles that support the pelvic organs, improving bladder and bowel control, and reducing the risk of prolapse. For seniors over 70, it's important to focus on exercises that are safe, effective, and can be done with minimal risk of injury. Here are seven pelvic floor exercises tailored for this age group, including the starting position, steps, repetitions, and their purpose:

1. Basic Kegels

- **Starting Position:** Sit comfortably in a chair or lie down on your back with knees bent and feet flat on the floor.
- **Steps:** Tighten your pelvic floor muscles as if you are trying to stop urine flow. Hold for 3-5 seconds, then relax for 3-5 seconds.
- **Repetitions:** Do 10-15 repetitions, 3 times a day.
- **Purpose:** Strengthens the pelvic floor muscles.

2. Seated Marches

- **Starting Position:** Sit in a chair with your feet flat on the ground, spine straight.
- **Steps:** Tighten your pelvic floor muscles. Lift one knee as if marching, place it down, and then lift the other knee. Keep your pelvic floor muscles engaged throughout.
- **Repetitions:** March for 1 minute. Rest, then repeat twice.
- **Purpose:** Engages and strengthens the pelvic floor along with improving lower body circulation.

3. Bridge

- **Starting Position:** Lie on your back with knees bent, feet flat on the floor, arms by your sides.
- **Steps:** Engage your pelvic floor muscles, then lift your hips towards the ceiling, forming a straight line from your knees to shoulders. Hold for 3-5 seconds, then slowly lower back down.
- **Repetitions:** Perform 10-15 bridges, rest, and repeat for 2 sets.
- **Purpose:** Strengthens the pelvic floor, glutes, and lower back.

4. Butterfly Stretch

- **Starting Position:** Sit on the floor, bend your knees to bring the soles of your feet together, and gently hold your feet with your hands.
- **Steps:** Keeping your back straight, gently press your knees down towards the floor as far as comfortable. You should feel a stretch, not pain.

- **Repetitions:** Hold the stretch for 30-45 seconds, relax, and repeat 3 times.
- **Purpose:** Improves flexibility and mobility in the pelvic area.

5. Leg Lifts

- **Starting Position:** Lie on your back with your legs straight and arms by your sides.
- **Steps:** Tighten your pelvic floor muscles. Slowly lift one leg a few inches off the ground, hold for a few seconds, then lower it. Repeat with the other leg.
- **Repetitions:** Do 10 lifts with each leg, rest, and then do another set.
- **Purpose:** Strengthens the pelvic floor and core muscles.

6. Wall Squats

- **Starting Position:** Stand with your back against a wall, feet shoulder-width apart.
- **Steps:** Engage your pelvic floor muscles, then slowly bend your knees to slide down the wall into a squat position. Hold for a few seconds, then slowly rise back up.
- **Repetitions:** Perform 8-10 squats, rest, and repeat for 2 sets.
- **Purpose:** Strengthens the pelvic floor, thighs, and buttocks.

7. Toe Taps

- **Starting Position:** Lie on your back with knees bent, feet lifted, and shins parallel to the floor.
- **Steps:** Tighten your pelvic floor muscles. Slowly tap one toe to the floor, then raise it back up. Alternate legs.
- **Repetitions:** Do 10 taps with each foot, rest, and repeat for 2 sets.
- **Purpose:** Engages the pelvic floor and lower abdominal muscles.

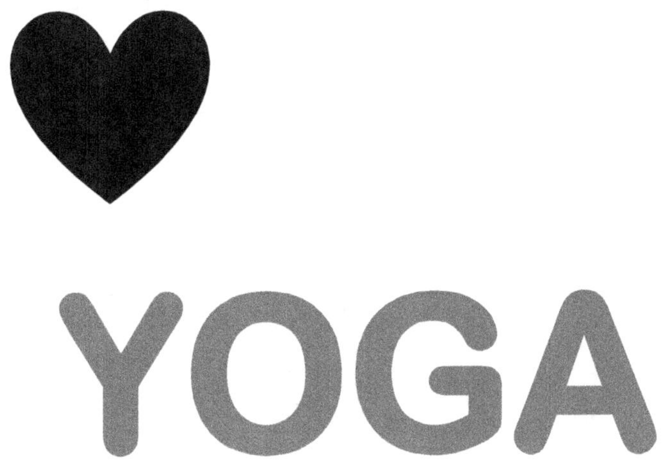

YOGA

TRACKER

<table>
<tr><td>DATE:</td><td>TIME:</td><td>BACK ☐</td><td>BICEPS ☐</td><td>LEGS ☐</td><td>ABS ☐</td></tr>
<tr><td colspan="2">M T W T F S S</td><td>CHEST ☐</td><td>TRICEPS ☐</td><td>CALVES ☐</td><td>OTHER ☐</td></tr>
<tr><td colspan="2"></td><td>CARDIO ☐</td><td>FOREARMS ☐</td><td colspan="2">SHOULDERS ☐</td></tr>
</table>

EXERCISE — 1 2 3 4 5 6 7 — WEIGHT

REPS	REPS	REPS	REPS	REPS	REPS

EXERCISE — 1 2 3 4 5 6 7 — WEIGHT

REPS	REPS	REPS	REPS	REPS	REPS

EXERCISE — 1 2 3 4 5 6 7 — WEIGHT

REPS	REPS	REPS	REPS	REPS	REPS

EXERCISE — 1 2 3 4 5 6 7 — WEIGHT

REPS	REPS	REPS	REPS	REPS	REPS

EXERCISE — 1 2 3 4 5 6 7 — WEIGHT

REPS	REPS	REPS	REPS	REPS	REPS

EXERCISE — 1 2 3 4 5 6 7 — WEIGHT

REPS	REPS	REPS	REPS	REPS	REPS

EXERCISE — 1 2 3 4 5 6 7 — WEIGHT

REPS	REPS	REPS	REPS	REPS	REPS

CARDIO	TIME	DIST.	PACE	INT.	HR
PRE-WORKOUT					
POST-WORKOUT					

DATE: TIME:

M T W T F S S

BACK ☐ BICEPS ☐ LEGS ☐ ABS ☐
CHEST ☐ TRICEPS ☐ CALVES ☐ OTHER ☐
CARDIO ☐ FOREARMS ☐ SHOULDERS ☐

EXERCISE	REPS	REPS	REPS	REPS	REPS	REPS
1 2 3 4 5 6 7 WEIGHT						

EXERCISE	REPS	REPS	REPS	REPS	REPS	REPS
1 **2** 3 4 5 6 7 WEIGHT						

EXERCISE	REPS	REPS	REPS	REPS	REPS	REPS
1 2 **3** 4 5 6 7 WEIGHT						

EXERCISE	REPS	REPS	REPS	REPS	REPS	REPS
1 2 3 **4** 5 6 7 WEIGHT						

EXERCISE	REPS	REPS	REPS	REPS	REPS	REPS
1 2 3 4 **5** 6 7 WEIGHT						

EXERCISE	REPS	REPS	REPS	REPS	REPS	REPS
1 2 3 4 5 **6** 7 WEIGHT						

EXERCISE	REPS	REPS	REPS	REPS	REPS	REPS
1 2 3 4 5 6 **7** WEIGHT						

CARDIO	TIME	DIST.	PACE	INT.	HR	
PRE-WORKOUT						
POST-WORKOUT						

DATE: TIME:

M T W T F S S

BACK ☐	BICEPS ☐	LEGS ☐	ABS ☐
CHEST ☐	TRICEPS ☐	CALVES ☐	OTHER ☐
CARDIO ☐	FOREARMS ☐	SHOULDERS ☐	

EXERCISE

1 2 3 4 5 6 7   WEIGHT

REPS ☐	REPS ☐	REPS ☐	REPS ☐	REPS ☐	REPS ☐

EXERCISE

1 **2** 3 4 5 6 7   WEIGHT

REPS ☐	REPS ☐	REPS ☐	REPS ☐	REPS ☐	REPS ☐

EXERCISE

1 2 **3** 4 5 6 7   WEIGHT

REPS ☐	REPS ☐	REPS ☐	REPS ☐	REPS ☐	REPS ☐

EXERCISE

1 2 3 **4** 5 6 7   WEIGHT

REPS ☐	REPS ☐	REPS ☐	REPS ☐	REPS ☐	REPS ☐

EXERCISE

1 2 3 4 **5** 6 7   WEIGHT

REPS ☐	REPS ☐	REPS ☐	REPS ☐	REPS ☐	REPS ☐

EXERCISE

1 2 3 4 5 **6** 7   WEIGHT

REPS ☐	REPS ☐	REPS ☐	REPS ☐	REPS ☐	REPS ☐

EXERCISE

1 2 3 4 5 6 **7**   WEIGHT

REPS ☐	REPS ☐	REPS ☐	REPS ☐	REPS ☐	REPS ☐

CARDIO

PRE-WORKOUT

POST-WORKOUT

TIME	DIST.	PACE	INT.	HR

DATE: | TIME:

M T W T F S S

BACK ☐ BICEPS ☐ LEGS ☐ ABS ☐
CHEST ☐ TRICEPS ☐ CALVES ☐ OTHER ☐
CARDIO ☐ FOREARMS ☐ SHOULDERS ☐

EXERCISE

1 2 3 4 5 6 7   WEIGHT

REPS	REPS	REPS	REPS	REPS	REPS

EXERCISE

1 **2** 3 4 5 6 7   WEIGHT

REPS	REPS	REPS	REPS	REPS	REPS

EXERCISE

1 2 **3** 4 5 6 7   WEIGHT

REPS	REPS	REPS	REPS	REPS	REPS

EXERCISE

1 2 3 **4** 5 6 7   WEIGHT

REPS	REPS	REPS	REPS	REPS	REPS

EXERCISE

1 2 3 4 **5** 6 7   WEIGHT

REPS	REPS	REPS	REPS	REPS	REPS

EXERCISE

1 2 3 4 5 **6** 7   WEIGHT

REPS	REPS	REPS	REPS	REPS	REPS

EXERCISE

1 2 3 4 5 6 **7**   WEIGHT

REPS	REPS	REPS	REPS	REPS	REPS

CARDIO

	TIME	DIST.	PACE	INT.	HR	
PRE-WORKOUT						
POST-WORKOUT						

DATE: TIME:

BACK ☐ BICEPS ☐ LEGS ☐ ABS ☐
CHEST ☐ TRICEPS ☐ CALVES ☐ OTHER ☐
CARDIO ☐ FOREARMS ☐ SHOULDERS ☐

| M | T | W | T | F | S | S |

EXERCISE

1 2 3 4 5 6 7   WEIGHT

REPS	REPS	REPS	REPS	REPS	REPS

EXERCISE

1 **2** 3 4 5 6 7   WEIGHT

REPS	REPS	REPS	REPS	REPS	REPS

EXERCISE

1 2 **3** 4 5 6 7   WEIGHT

REPS	REPS	REPS	REPS	REPS	REPS

EXERCISE

1 2 3 **4** 5 6 7   WEIGHT

REPS	REPS	REPS	REPS	REPS	REPS

EXERCISE

1 2 3 4 **5** 6 7   WEIGHT

REPS	REPS	REPS	REPS	REPS	REPS

EXERCISE

1 2 3 4 5 **6** 7   WEIGHT

REPS	REPS	REPS	REPS	REPS	REPS

EXERCISE

1 2 3 4 5 6 **7**   WEIGHT

REPS	REPS	REPS	REPS	REPS	REPS

CARDIO

PRE-WORKOUT

POST-WORKOUT

TIME	DIST.	PACE	INT.	HR	

DATE: TIME:

M **T** **W** **T** **F** **S** **S**

BACK ☐   BICEPS ☐   LEGS ☐   ABS ☐
CHEST ☐   TRICEPS ☐   CALVES ☐   OTHER ☐
CARDIO ☐   FOREARMS ☐   SHOULDERS ☐

EXERCISE	REPS	REPS	REPS	REPS	REPS	REPS
1 234567 WEIGHT						

EXERCISE	REPS	REPS	REPS	REPS	REPS	REPS
1 **2** 34567 WEIGHT						

EXERCISE	REPS	REPS	REPS	REPS	REPS	REPS
12 **3** 4567 WEIGHT						

EXERCISE	REPS	REPS	REPS	REPS	REPS	REPS
123 **4** 567 WEIGHT						

EXERCISE	REPS	REPS	REPS	REPS	REPS	REPS
1234 **5** 67 WEIGHT						

EXERCISE	REPS	REPS	REPS	REPS	REPS	REPS
12345 **6** 7 WEIGHT						

EXERCISE	REPS	REPS	REPS	REPS	REPS	REPS
123456 **7** WEIGHT						

CARDIO	TIME	DIST.	PACE	INT.	HR	
PRE-WORKOUT						
POST-WORKOUT						

DATE: TIME:

M **T** **W** **T** **F** **S** **S**

BACK ☐   BICEPS ☐   LEGS ☐   ABS ☐
CHEST ☐   TRICEPS ☐   CALVES ☐   OTHER ☐
CARDIO ☐   FOREARMS ☐   SHOULDERS ☐

EXERCISE	REPS	REPS	REPS	REPS	REPS	REPS
1 2 3 4 5 6 7 WEIGHT						

EXERCISE	REPS	REPS	REPS	REPS	REPS	REPS
1 **2** 3 4 5 6 7 WEIGHT						

EXERCISE	REPS	REPS	REPS	REPS	REPS	REPS
1 2 **3** 4 5 6 7 WEIGHT						

EXERCISE	REPS	REPS	REPS	REPS	REPS	REPS
1 2 3 **4** 5 6 7 WEIGHT						

EXERCISE	REPS	REPS	REPS	REPS	REPS	REPS
1 2 3 4 **5** 6 7 WEIGHT						

EXERCISE	REPS	REPS	REPS	REPS	REPS	REPS
1 2 3 4 5 **6** 7 WEIGHT						

EXERCISE	REPS	REPS	REPS	REPS	REPS	REPS
1 2 3 4 5 6 **7** WEIGHT						

CARDIO	TIME	DIST.	PACE	INT.	HR	
PRE-WORKOUT						
POST-WORKOUT						

DATE: | TIME:

M T W T F S S

BACK ☐   BICEPS ☐   LEGS ☐   ABS ☐
CHEST ☐   TRICEPS ☐   CALVES ☐   OTHER ☐
CARDIO ☐   FOREARMS ☐   SHOULDERS ☐

EXERCISE	REPS	REPS	REPS	REPS	REPS	REPS
1 234567 WEIGHT						

EXERCISE	REPS	REPS	REPS	REPS	REPS	REPS
1 **2** 34567 WEIGHT						

EXERCISE	REPS	REPS	REPS	REPS	REPS	REPS
12 **3** 4567 WEIGHT						

EXERCISE	REPS	REPS	REPS	REPS	REPS	REPS
123 **4** 567 WEIGHT						

EXERCISE	REPS	REPS	REPS	REPS	REPS	REPS
1234 **5** 67 WEIGHT						

EXERCISE	REPS	REPS	REPS	REPS	REPS	REPS
12345 **6** 7 WEIGHT						

EXERCISE	REPS	REPS	REPS	REPS	REPS	REPS
123456 **7** WEIGHT						

CARDIO	TIME	DIST.	PACE	INT.	HR	
PRE-WORKOUT						
POST-WORKOUT						

DATE: TIME:

M T W T F S S

BACK ☐ BICEPS ☐ LEGS ☐ ABS ☐
CHEST ☐ TRICEPS ☐ CALVES ☐ OTHER ☐
CARDIO ☐ FOREARMS ☐ SHOULDERS ☐

EXERCISE	REPS	REPS	REPS	REPS	REPS	REPS
1 2 3 4 5 6 7 WEIGHT						
EXERCISE	REPS	REPS	REPS	REPS	REPS	REPS
1 **2** 3 4 5 6 7 WEIGHT						
EXERCISE	REPS	REPS	REPS	REPS	REPS	REPS
1 2 **3** 4 5 6 7 WEIGHT						
EXERCISE	REPS	REPS	REPS	REPS	REPS	REPS
1 2 3 **4** 5 6 7 WEIGHT						
EXERCISE	REPS	REPS	REPS	REPS	REPS	REPS
1 2 3 4 **5** 6 7 WEIGHT						
EXERCISE	REPS	REPS	REPS	REPS	REPS	REPS
1 2 3 4 5 **6** 7 WEIGHT						
EXERCISE	REPS	REPS	REPS	REPS	REPS	REPS
1 2 3 4 5 6 **7** WEIGHT						

CARDIO	TIME	DIST.	PACE	INT.	HR	
PRE-WORKOUT						
POST-WORKOUT